THE TEMPER
FOR WOMEN

KU-694-779

THE TEMPERATURE GUIDE
FOR WOMEN

by

DR SACHA GELLER

With a Foreword by
Dr John Marshall

and a Preface by
Professor Max Jayle

LONDON
BURNS & OATES

This translation of La Température Guide de la Femme
(René Julliard, Paris) was made by a Catholic doctor

NIHIL OBSTAT : JOANNES M. T. BARTON, S.T.D., L.S.S.

CENSOR DEPUTATUS

IMPRIMATUR : ✠ GEORGIUS L. CRAVEN

EPISCOPUS SEBASTOPOLIS

VIC. CAP.

WESTMONASTERII : DIE Iᴀ MARTII 1963

The Nihil obstat *and* Imprimatur *are a declaration that a book or pamphlet is considered to be free from doctrinal or moral error. It is not implied that those who have granted the* Nihil obstat *and* Imprimatur *agree with the contents, opinions or statements expressed.*

© René Julliard 1960

English translation © Burns & Oates Ltd 1964
Catalogue No.: 5/5147

MADE AND PRINTED IN GREAT BRITAIN BY
BILLING AND SONS LIMITED, GUILDFORD AND LONDON
FOR BURNS AND OATES LIMITED, 25 ASHLEY PLACE, LONDON, S.W.1

FOREWORD

by DR JOHN MARSHALL

THE spectacular advances in medical science of the last quarter of a century in antibiotic therapy, cardiac surgery and vaccination against poliomyelitis, to mention but a few, have overshadowed the less spectacular, but no less important, progress in the understanding of the cycle of fertility and infertility in woman. Some awareness of this cycle has existed since biblical times, but the knowledge was too vague to be of practical value. That this should have remained the case for so long is surprising in view of the amount of ill health, anxiety and misery caused by failure to regulate conception and the size of the family in accordance with its needs and resources. It becomes more surprising when we consider the widely recognized aesthetic and psychological objections to contraceptive methods of regulation, objections which pose an insurmountable barrier to many married people. Nor has the introduction of oral methods of contraception relieved this situation, for many people are disturbed about the use of a drug which so profoundly disrupts female reproductive physiology. The development of a method of regulating the size of the family which does not involve interference with the act of intercourse nor with human physiology, and which is, moreover, acceptable to those whose ethical beliefs lead them to oppose other methods, is long overdue.

The pioneer work of Ogino and Knaus provided a sound basis for such a development, but, as Dr Geller shows in this book, further refinement was necessary.

This has been provided by the method of recording the basal temperature. By this means the fertile and infertile times of the cycle can be determined with such accuracy as to provide a practical means of regulating the size of the family. Not only is the method reliable when properly applied, but it can serve to enhance and deepen marital experience. The necessary discipline prevents intercourse from ever becoming the automatic response to physical urges, and fulfilment is the greater for having been, by mutual consent, delayed.

There can be no doubt that there has in the past been much dissatisfaction and even disillusionment with the use of the infertile period as a means of regulating the size of the family. Study of these pages quickly shows why, for it is clear that much of the advice tendered to married people was not in accordance with the best physiological knowledge accumulated over the last three decades. Dr Geller's profound understanding of this problem and his extensive practical experience in guiding married people has enabled him to produce a book which is both scientifically valid, and simply and lucidly written. It will undoubtedly bring great help to countless married people who desire to regulate the size of their family without destroying the beauty of the most significant of human acts.

CONTENTS

PART ONE

REPRODUCTIVE LIFE OF WOMAN AND TEMPERATURE CURVE

PART TWO

PREFACE

by PROFESSOR MAX JAYLE

WHEN reaffirming the adoption by the Church of the method of periodic abstention, which alone can reconcile the precepts of the Faith with the legitimate needs of the individual, Pope Pius XII expressed the hope that medical science "might succeed in giving a sufficiently solid basis for this permissible method".[1]

Dr Geller's book has come to give concrete expression to this hope.

One knows how divided opinions have been with regard to the laws formulated by Ogino and Knaus (O.K.). Optimists give them the "O.K." and place all their confidence in them. Pessimists see in them the best means of populating desert lands!

Between these two extreme positions one should recognize that the Ogino-Knaus method, the first stage in the liberation of woman, has rendered unquestionable service and still does so; but it is liable to certain misconceptions. These, as Dr Geller shows, depend upon the hypothetical nature of the calculations as to ovulation which are postulated by this method.

In order to render this method of periodic abstention sufficiently sure, and to give it a solid basis, it was necessary to have a precise and accurate index of the date of ovulation in the cycle. Once the date of ovulation could be fixed by the changes in the temperature, thanks chiefly to the work of Palmer in France, the

[1] *Acta Apostolica Sedis*, Vol. XVIII, p. 859. Pontifical addresses No. 204, Allocution to Associations of Large Families, p. 389, n. 667.

thermal curve has been used to determine with greater accuracy on which days in the cycle a woman is liable to be fertilized. But it has needed the possibility of hormonal investigation to be able to render a valid interpretation of all the information given by the thermal curve. Being both an expert clinician and well versed in endocrine investigations, Dr Geller, thanks to his double orientation, has been able to grasp in all its subtlety, and to prove the remarkable accuracy, of this very simple procedure.

But, in order to make judicious use of it, it is essential to have a sound knowledge of its basis. It was therefore necessary to give the lay public some idea of the knowledge which we have of ovarian physiology. In this scientific introduction to the subject Dr Geller shows himself to be a gifted writer, and has been able to explain biological facts in a way which makes for attractive reading. We shall see that the author has succeeded in his task of making the complex mechanisms subserving the development of the menstrual cycle understandable to all.

From now on, *every woman* can, with the minimum of effort, understand the method, derive the maximum profit from it, and also understand its limits.

Through this increased understanding of the secrets of their physiology, women can now space births for the greater harmony of the home. For couples who are not adequately fertile it will be possible to ensure the best conditions for pregnancy, seeking if necessary the help of the doctor. From this point of view this book will be of great assistance to gynaecologists.

We no longer live in an age when a female patient in China showed her doctor the location of her troubles on a little ivory figure. Methods of investigating functions have provided medicine with the means of measuring the activity of organs. This does not only mean the collaboration between a specialist and a well-equipped laboratory; it is equally necessary that the patient should herself contribute, because investigations must be carried out at certain precise moments during the menstrual cycle established by means of the thermal curve. By giving to every woman a practical physiological guide, Dr Geller has done valuable service.

By the light which it sheds upon the workings of the genital system, and by the knowledge which it can impart to a woman in respect of her physiological profile, Dr Geller's book also contributes to the emancipation of the individual. It is in line with that train of thought already adumbrated by Alexis Carrel in *Man, the Unknown*, where he states his conviction that the biological sciences are not for doctors and scientists alone, but have a role to play in upholding the dignity of modern man, who must be conscious of his physiological functions in order to acquire greater control over his health and well-being. Thus the knowledge given by the science of biology links up with the wisdom of the ancients: "know thyself". By rendering the transmission of life a conscious act, this knowledge harmonizes perfectly with the highest philosophical concepts.

This little book can therefore play a very important educative role, whether in helping a young woman with her periods of maternity, which she can harmonize with the economic needs of her home, or of allowing her to provide her doctor with all the information which he requires in order to look after her better. The author of this book deserves the thanks and congratulations of all those women who will not fail to benefit by it; not only for themselves, but for the moral and physical well-being of their home.

INTRODUCTION

IN these days, when a woman consults her doctor for ovarian trouble, he may well ask her to note her temperature curve. Not because he suspects some infection, but because it is a well-known fact that the temperature, taken under certain conditions, can give valuable information about the function of the ovaries.

This remarkable property of the temperature curve, suspected from the beginning of this century by the Dutch physician Van de Velde, and the French gynaecologist Fruhinsholz, was experimentally demonstrated twenty years or so ago by the work of Rubenstein and Zuck in America, and especially by that of Palmer in France, to which we owe the essential knowledge which we now have of the subject.

Doctors who use the temperature curve, which is now well established in medical practice, know what valuable information with regard both to diagnosis and treatment of ovarian disorders it provides.

It appears to us, however, that every woman should find it to her interest to get to know her temperature tracing, and it is the object of this book to enable her to acquire this knowledge. The regulation of births is certainly of paramount interest to the woman; the temperature curve provides a sure and simple means of determining for herself on which days of the cycle she may become pregnant, and which not.

Since no one today would seriously deny the right of every married woman to space births in a reasonable manner, it would seem only right to place within her reach a simple, and above all natural, solution to a problem which can be agonizing. In this way she can knowingly embark upon a pregnancy which has been desired and sought for, and avoid the spectre of one which is, at least temporarily, undesired and inopportune.

But to regard this work merely as a series of practical formulas would be to restrict its significance and range quite unjustifiably. On account of its simplicity and accuracy, the temperature curve gives us a most valuable means of getting to know and to observe the nature of the menstrual cycle up to its natural issue, pregnancy; and thus to follow and control the whole sexual life of woman from puberty to menopause. Thus the temperature curve renders it possible for every woman to acquire a knowledge and become conscious of what might be termed her physiological self, which will certainly be of great benefit to her.

PART ONE

REPRODUCTIVE LIFE OF WOMAN
AND TEMPERATURE CURVE

1

THE MENSTRUAL CYCLE

WHAT woman has not pondered, at one time or another, on the mystery of menstruation, and the reasons for this "eternal return"?

Such a striking phenomenon could not fail to impress people's minds, and from olden times menstruation has given rise to many different beliefs, mainly connected with ideas of impurity. Thus among the Jews, if we are to believe the tradition, it was held that a woman is impure during the whole time of menstruation, and for the week following; among Gypsies a woman in this state cannot prepare the man's food without sullying it. Even in our day women attribute a "purgative" role to menstruation: as though the "peccant humours", dear to physicians of old, were thus eliminated.

In fact, as we know today, menstruation is but an index of the reproductive cycle: with each "period" commences a cycle of events which renders it possible for the female organism to procreate. With each cycle indeed the female ripens and liberates a reproductive cell, the ovum, the fertilization of which will result in the formation of a human foetus. Such is the general significance of the female cycle, which develops in phases from one menstrual period to another.

THE OVARY, A STORE-HOUSE OF FOLLICLES

Nature has supplied woman with a generous provision of ova, which are carefully kept in reserve in the interior of the sexual glands, the ovaries. These are almond-shaped bodies with a somewhat embossed

3

B

surface, the interior of which is literally stuffed with
ova. Each ovary contains about 300,000 of them, of
which only between 300 and 400 at the most will be
shed during the whole reproductive life of the female,
and of these but a few will be fertilized. That is to say
that every precaution is taken in order that there may
be no failure of the primary material![1]

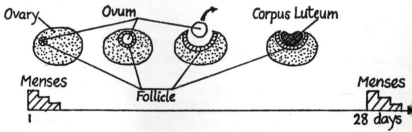

FIG. 1 : *Maturation of the ovum*

Shows the ovary with one follicle and its ovum at different
stages of the menstrual cycle.

(*a*) At the beginning of the cycle, the follicle is small.

(*b*) The follicle has grown and is nearing the surface of the
ovary.

(*c*) Towards the 14th day, the follicle is ripe, reaches the surface of the ovary, bursts out, and discharges the contained ovum.

(*d*) After the ovum has left, a "yellow body" (corpus luteum)
is formed in the ruptured follicle.

THE MATURATION OF THE OVUM

Let us now look a little more closely at the process
of maturation of the ovum (Fig. 1).

Each ovum is surrounded by a small covering, the
follicle, which develops conjointly. This is very small at
the beginning of the cycle, and as it grows it approaches

[1] Nature shows herself no less generous with the male: in
the course of a single act of coitus between three and four
hundred million sperms are set free, and of these only one will
fertilize the ovum. Such is the prodigality of means to ensure
the propagation of species.

the surface of the ovary. Having achieved a state of sufficient maturity, towards the 14th day of the cycle, the follicle will reach the surface of the ovary where it will burst, like a ripe fruit, and liberate the ovum which is contained in it: this is what is meant by *ovulation*, which is in fact but the last stage in the maturation of the follicle with its ovum.

ODYSSEY OF THE OVUM

Once freed, the ovum has not yet reached its goal: to get to the place which Nature has ordained, it must pass into the genital tract (Fig. 2).

With this end in view, the fallopian tube, which has an orifice at the tip for the passage of the ovum, is carried towards the ovary, rather like a tentacle, and literally swallows the ovum, which is engulfed in it (Fig. 2, square). Once in place, the ovum has only to await the coming of the sperm which is to fertilize it. For it is within the tube that fertilization will take place, and the sperms put into the vagina during intercourse ascend the genital tract to meet the ovum (Fig. 2, arrows).

Of the myriad sperms which seek to conquer the ovum, only one, the most vigorous of them, will enter the ovum and fertilize it.[1]

The ovum which is thus fertilized will now form the initial cell of the egg. This will be transported by the movements of the tube into the uterine cavity, where it will become fixed and where it will develop. For this purpose the uterine cavity is covered with an interior lining like that of a garment, the *uterine mucosa* (Fig. 2), in which the ovum becomes embedded, and through

---

[1] The other sperms are not useless, however. They produce a ferment which strips the ovum and thus renders it easier for the sperm to enter it.

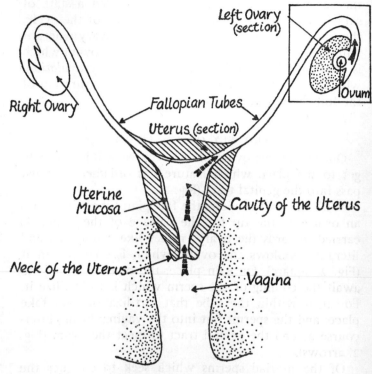

FIG. 2 : *Female genital organs*

Including, from below upwards : (1) *Vagina*; (2) *Cavity of the uterus*, a hollow organ, in the shape of a pear reversed; the tip or uterine cervix opening into the top of the vaginal cavity. The inside of the uterus is lined by the uterine mucosa; (3) The *fallopian tubes*, narrow conduits which prolong the uterine cavity on each side, and come into contact with the corresponding ovary.

The square on the right side shows the ovary in section, with the end of the tube, and the orifice through which the ovum proceeds in the course of ovulation.

The black arrow shows the route of the ovum; the dotted arrows, that followed by the sperms.

which it will receive from the maternal organism the nourishment which is necessary for its development.

It is as though the ovum had need of the sperm in order to survive; as though this embrace brought to it the elixir of life. In fact if it is not fertilized, if it has waited in vain, the ovum will only survive for a few hours—12 to 24 at the most—after ovulation. After this interval it rapidly degenerates and dies.

Let us now come back to the ovary, from where we started.

The Corpus Luteum

Whether the ovum be fertilized or not, important changes are going on in the interior of the follicle which has just been vacated by the ovum. After it has gone, a yellowish material, known for this reason as the "corpus luteum", is formed in the cavity of the follicle (Fig. 1*d*).

This body is an endocrine gland[1] which secretes a hormone as soon as it is formed. It is carried by the blood to the uterine mucosa to prepare it for the possible pregnancy. This is done by accumulating there the nutritive substances needed in the first stages of development of the ovum which has been shed and fertilized. The uterine mucosa, which is thin before ovulation, thickens and increases under the influence of the hormone provided by the corpus luteum; just as grass will grow when it is watered (Fig. 3*a*, *b*). Thus, without knowing whether or not the ovum will be fertilized, the corpus luteum, with its hormonal secretion, prepares as it were a "nuptial couch" in which the ovum will come to lie.

---

[1] An endocrine gland is built up of cells which have the power to secrete certain substances which are then passed into the blood vessels. These substances are called *hormones* and are carried by the blood stream into other organs, the function of which they can influence, or the growth of which they can stimulate.

MENSTRUATION

Should the egg not be fertilized, all these preparations are rendered useless. As though forewarned in some mysterious manner, the corpus luteum stops secreting at the end of 14 days or, in general, not less than 12 or more than 16 days after ovulation has occurred.[1]

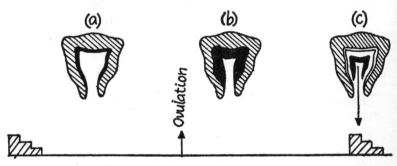

FIG. 3: *Mechanism of menstruation*

The uterus is shown (in section) covered by the mucous membrane (in black) at different times of the cycle.

(*a*) Before ovulation, the mucosa is thin.

(*b*) After ovulation, the mucosa thickens and increases under the influence of the hormones of the corpus luteum which has appeared after ovulation.

(*c*) The superficial part of the uterine mucosa, which is no longer nourished by the hormones of the corpus luteum, separates, causing the bleeding of menstruation.

Then the uterine mucosa, deprived of hormonal nourishment, will wither like a leaf without sap, and its superficial layer is loosened, taking with it the now useless materials: this separation leaves a bare surface and from this flows the blood which constitutes the menses (Fig. 3*c*). Menstrual bleeding will not stop until the

[1] This cessation is brought about automatically by a complex process, which is comparable to a thermostat in a frigidaire or hot water tank, which breaks the contact when the required temperature is reached.

wound is quite healed and this usually takes from 3 to 6 days.[1]

THE SUCCESSIVE CYCLES

The appearance of menstruation marks the beginning of a new cycle. Another follicle will become mature and liberate its ovum; once more a corpus luteum will form, and its hormones will prepare the uterine mucosa for a possible pregnancy. In the absence of fertilization, once again the hormonal secretion of the corpus luteum will cease, precipitating the appearance of the next menstrual cycle, and so on: *thus untiringly with each cycle, the female organism prepares itself in the hope of pregnancy.*

From this somewhat deterministic point of view the woman, with her menstrual cycle, is seen as the more or less conscious instrument of a mysterious creative force, and menstruation as the expression of the "uterine deception".

THE TWO PHASES OF THE MENSTRUAL CYCLE

In studying the development of the menstrual cycle, it will be seen that it consists of two successive phases (Fig. 4).

(a) The first, which extends from the first day of the cycle until ovulation occurs, is given up to the maturation of the follicle and its ovum: this is the *follicular phase* which ends with ovulation.

Its usual duration is about 14 *days, but it may be shorter, or more often, it may be prolonged beyond the* 14 *days,* when the process of maturation is impaired: in this case, of course, ovulation will take place more or less later than the 14th day of the cycle.

---

[1] The menses therefore correspond simply with a bared surface which heals more or less quickly. Thus the last day of the "period" has no special significance. This is why the cycle must be estimated from the first day of the menses.

(*b*) Following ovulation begins the second phase, which is characterized by the presence of the corpus luteum; for this reason it is called the *luteal phase*. This phase extends from the ovulation to the end of the cycle; that is to say, till the onset of the following menstruation.

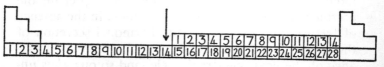

FIG. 4: *The two phases of the menstrual cycle*

The follicular phase extends from the 1st day of the cycle (which is the 1st day of the period) until the ovulation (marked by the arrow) which finishes it.

The luteal phase starts immediately following this and continues to the end of the cycle.

Its normal duration is also about 14 *days,* since this is the average duration of the corpus luteum. *But in contrast to the follicular phase, the luteal phase cannot last longer than* 16 *days.*

We have already seen that if in fact the ovum is not fertilized, the corpus luteum ceases to secrete, and menstruation follows inevitably after a period of 16 days at most, after ovulation, corresponding to the maximum duration of the corpus luteum.[1]

[1] Ovulation having in a sense been "missed", it is important that menstruation should supervene, in order that a fresh ovum be brought to maturity and thus offer a fresh chance of pregnancy. This end is attained by the cessation of the hormone secretion of the corpus luteum, the life of which must therefore be compulsorily limited.

2

THE FERTILE AND STERILE DAYS
OF THE CYCLE:
THE LAWS OF OGINO-KNAUS

THE idea that women are only fertile at certain times of the menstrual cycle seems to have been suspected, even if not definitely known, since ancient times, if one can judge from customs, traditions, or religious rites.

The explanation of this phenomenon, however, was only discovered when it became known that the cycle involved ovulation: it then became clear that a woman could only be fertilized at the time of ovulation, since this was the only opportunity for the sperm to meet the ovum and fertilize it.

It could then be supposed that it would suffice to know the date at which ovulation occurred during the cycle in order to deduce the fertile and sterile days within the cycle.

Thus, at the beginning of the century, various investigators tried to determine by various methods[1] the date of ovulation in the cycle.

Unfortunately the first researches showed an extraordinary discrepancy in their results as between different workers: for some, ovulation occurred between the 14th and 16th days of the cycle, for others between the 11th and 18th, for yet others between the 8th and 21st; there were some even who thought that ovulation might occur at any day of the cycle.

---

[1] Notably by studying pregnancies which followed upon intercourse on given days of the cycle.

In fact it seemed that ovulation was very variable, and that no prevision was possible, so that the question of the determination of fertile and sterile days appeared insoluble.

Then towards 1930 Knaus in Germany and Ogino in Japan made observations of great importance which were to clarify the situation considerably.

The method which they proposed had the great merit of offering a solution, however imperfect as yet, to this vexing problem.

We will therefore explain the method briefly before criticizing it, and considering the fresh solution offered by the thermal curve.

THE OBSERVATIONS OF OGINO-KNAUS

Like their predecessors, Ogino and Knaus were trying to determine the date of ovulation, and for this they employed different methods. Ogino, who was a surgeon, examined the ovaries of women upon whom he had operated at different stages of the menstrual cycle. Knaus, whose work lay in biology, studied the contractions of the uterus to certain stimuli with hormones, by means of an ingenious experimental technique. Since the uterus did not respond to the stimulus after ovulation, Knaus could devise a method whereby he was able to register the date of ovulation with accuracy.

Although working separately, the two came to much the same conclusions almost simultaneously; like their predecessors, they found the dates of ovulation to be variable according to the different cycles which they investigated. But they had a flash of inspiration, which was to count the dates of ovulation, not from the preceding periods, but backwards; that is starting from the next expected period.

They then made the following surprising observation: whatever the type of menstrual cycle, ovulation never occurred nearer than 12 days and never further than 16 days from the onset of the next menses. Whatever the length of the cycle, *ovulation is therefore produced between the 16th and 12th day preceding the onset of the next menstrual period* (Fig. 5).

SIGNIFICANCE OF THE OBSERVATIONS

That there is an interval of 12 to 16 days between ovulation and the menstrual period which follows, no longer looks strange to us since we now know that between ovulation and the end of the cycle there is the corpus luteum, the duration of which varies from a minimum of 12 days to a maximum of 16 (see p. 8).

This mysterious interval between ovulation and the

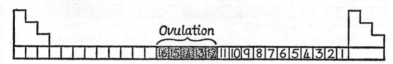

FIG. 5: *Observations of Ogino-Knaus*

menstruation which follows corresponds, therefore, simply to the duration of the cyclic corpus luteum.

It was logical enough, as we now realize, to tie up ovulation, not to the menses which precede it, but to those that follow it, since the latter represent the end result of a chain of events (formation of the corpus luteum, hormonal secretion of the corpus, and cessation of this secretion) which have been started off with ovulation.

FERTILE AND STERILE PERIODS OF THE CYCLE

The observations of Ogino and Knaus were bound to create a considerable impression, because they made it possible to define those periods in the cycle when a woman either was or was not liable to fertilization.

According to the preceding observations in fact, *starting from the menstrual period which is to come*, and working back to the beginning of the cycle, we find first of all a sterile period represented by the 11 last days of the cycle, and this is the *terminal sterile ("safe") period* (Fig. 6).

The 5 days beyond that period, i.e. 12th, 13th, 14th, 15th and 16th days counting back from the expected period, *are those days of the cycle when ovulation is likely to occur*. These five days obviously pertain to the fertile period of the cycle; but this period extends be-

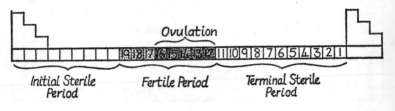

FIG. 6: *Fertile and sterile periods of the cycle* (explained in the text)

yond these five days because of the possible survival of the sperm.

It must be understood in fact that whereas the ovum which is not fertilized will degenerate in a few hours, the sperms on the other hand are more resistant, and can still survive for one or two days. So intercourse on the eve of, or the day before, the earliest ovulation can still prove to be fertile. If it is desired to avoid pregnancy therefore, it is necessary to abstain during both of the two days preceding ovulation, i.e. the 17th, the 18th, and, for greater security still, the 19th day before the expected menstrual period. *The fertile period therefore extends from the 12th to the 19th day before the expected menstrual period* (Fig. 6).

Beyond this fertile period there is another sterile period: this is *the initial sterile ("safe") period*, which corresponds to those days which are left when the last nineteen days have been taken off from the whole cycle (Fig. 6).

THE OGINO-KNAUS CALCULATION

If one knew the length of the cycle in advance, it would be easy to determine which are the "available" days in the cycle. From what has just been said it follows that one would merely take away 19 days from the duration of the cycle to obtain the number of days which are "safe" at the beginning of the cycle. After this, it would be a matter of abstaining until the 12th day before the end of the cycle, which is easily obtained by taking away 11 days from its end.

Example: In a cycle fixed at 28 days, one would have at the beginning of the cycle $28 - 19 = 9$ days, then there would be a period of abstention until the $(28 - 11)$, i.e. the 17th day of the cycle.

It is true that one does not know in advance the exact length of the cycle. Nevertheless one can presume that it will be comprised between the shortest and the longest cycles hitherto observed.

Now, according to this calculation, the shorter the cycle the more the initial sterile ("safe") period is reduced. On the other hand, the longer the cycle the longer does the period of abstention take to finish.

If, therefore, one is to allow for all possibilities in the forthcoming cycle, between the shortest and longest, the initial sterile period must be calculated from the shortest cycle, and the period of abstention from the longest. Hence, in order to calculate the initial sterile period, *the 19 days must be taken from the length of the SHORTEST cycle* previously observed; and, to calculate the end of the period of abstention, 11 days *must be taken away from the LONGEST cycle pre-viously observed.*[1]

Example: Suppose a cycle which varies between 26 and 32 days. At the beginning of the cycle there is available an initial sterile period of $26 - 19 = 7$ days. Abstention must then be observed until the $(32 - 11)$, i.e. 21st day of the cycle inclusive.

CONCLUSION

In short, there is a first sterile (or safe) period at the beginning of the cycle, the extent of which is dependent on the shortest cycle.

After this, there is a period of continence or abstention, the length of which depends on the longest cycle, and after which intercourse can be resumed. Such is, essentially, the principle of calculation laid down by Ogino-Knaus, and it is now necessary to discuss its validity.

---

[1] In order to determine the longest and shortest cycles, Ogino and Knaus advised that the menstrual cycle should be studied for at least a year.

3

CRITICISM OF THE METHOD OF OGINO-KNAUS

IT must be acknowledged that the Ogino-Knaus method has rendered and continues to render considerable service. Still, it is common knowledge that it has given rise to certain misconceptions, which have in fact tended to discredit it.

Although some of these are due to wrong application of its principles for which it is not responsible, there are some errors inherent in the very method; the calculation of Ogino is indeed an estimate of probability. As such it may prove to be wrong, and what we now know about the menstrual cycle will enable us to understand why and under what circumstances this will be the case.

THE FIRST STERILE PERIOD

We have seen that in order to calculate the first sterile period we must start from the *shortest cycle* previously determined, and that we take away 19 days from its duration. But immediately an objection may occur to us: what is to guarantee that there will not be a *still shorter cycle* than that which has been taken as a base-line?

It is true that a shortening of the cycle may be produced if the time of ovulation is advanced. In this case the sterile period at the beginning of the cycle is also shortened and intercourse at this time may result in pregnancy. Theoretically this danger cannot be denied. But, *in practice*, the danger is far less than might be supposed.

We have seen in fact that ovulation is the last stage

in the maturation of the ovum. From this it follows that in order to attain a successful result, i.e. the setting free of a fertilizable ovum, this process requires a certain duration. Experience shows that *at least* 8 *to* 10 *days are necessary for the ovum to ripen properly*.

No doubt it does happen, especially at the pre-menopausal period, when the ovarian function is declining and can no longer bring to its conclusion the maturation of the ovum, that ovulation may occur before the 10th day of the cycle. But, as a rule, the freed ovum in this case has not achieved sufficient maturity and is not capable of being fertilized. So that the danger of premature ovulation is practically negligible, and the calculation of the first sterile period has little chance of being in error.

The risk is all the less seeing that *the calculation is made under the least favourable conditions*: presupposing a corpus luteum of 16 days' duration, though the usual one is of 14 days only; moreover, where 2 extra days of abstention would have sufficed to counteract the possible survival of the sperm, this calculation as an extra precaution has demanded 3.

For all these reasons, *the calculation of Ogino relating to the first sterile period can be regarded as sufficiently reliable*. The same cannot be said, however, when we consider the determination of the end of the abstention period.

THE END OF THE PERIOD OF ABSTENTION

It must be remembered that, according to Ogino, the end of the period of abstention is to be calculated according to the longest cycle, and corresponds to the 12th day before the end of the cycle.

There is evidently no assurance that there may not be *an even longer cycle* in the future than the one which formed the basis of calculation. In this case, the period of abstention which is to be observed will end later, so that in resuming intercourse on the date previously permissible according to this method, it will still come into the fertile period and pregnancy may result.

Let us suppose that during the course of a year the cycles observed have not lasted more than 30 days. There is no reason why there may not supervene a cycle, for example, of 35 days. Now, in the 30-day cycle the period of abstention extended until the (30 − 11), i.e. 19th day of the cycle, which allowed for the resumption of intercourse from the 20th day. But in a cycle of 35 days the period of abstention should be prolonged until the (35 − 11), i.e. 24th day of the cycle. In this cycle, therefore, intercourse may be fertile until the 24th day. As one does not know in advance that the cycle may last 35 days, if intercourse is resumed from the 20th day, as was allowable by the method up to now, it is quite possible, obviously, that pregnancy may result.

Thus the possible lengthening of the cycle completely upsets the calculations according to Ogino. Since the interval between ovulation and the end of a cycle cannot be prolonged beyond 16 days, the lengthening of the cycle cannot be due to anything but a delayed ovulation. Hence it is the possible delay of ovulation which upsets calculations: *in resuming intercourse from the date allowed by the method, there is always the risk of lighting upon a delayed ovulation.*[1]

Now whereas, as we have seen, the risk of premature ovulation is very slight, that of delayed ovulation is very important.

---

[1] This is the explanation in particular of pregnancies which occur after a single intercourse immediately previous to the expected menses (which would have been delayed had there been no pregnancy).

C

This will be easily understood if it is recalled that ovulation is the final stage in the process of maturation. If there should be some hindrance to its development, the process will be slowed down, and ovulation will therefore be delayed. This is familiar to women who have observed how menstruation may be delayed or even stopped following a violent emotion, a cold bath, a journey, or even a simple change of climate. The process of ovulation is indeed governed by such complex and subtle factors that even a slight stimulus may upset its working. Ovulation is then suspended or postponed until the organism has resumed its normal working.

This eventuality is far from unusual, indeed common. Moreover, the duration of this blocking may vary. It follows that, no matter how long the period over which one has observed the duration of the menstrual cycles, and whatever the margin of safety adopted accordingly, there is no guarantee against the risk of delayed ovulation.

It is important to note that in the case of these retarded ovulations the maturation of the ovum may be perfectly in order, apart from the longer time which it has taken; the ovum thus liberated is perfectly fertilizable, contrary to what is the case in premature ovulation. Delay in ovulation therefore brings undoubted risks of pregnancy; this is a frequent and unpredictable occurrence. *The delay in ovulation is indeed the stumbling-block in the method of Ogino-Knaus, which gives no protection against this major risk.*[1]

---

[1] In this connection the list of circumstances in which, according to the advocates of the Ogino-Knaus method themselves, it may not be used is significant: illness, after childbirth or a miscarriage, while breast-feeding or weaning, travelling, change of climate, change of diet or way of life (!), irregularities caused by the menopause, etc.

SHORT DURATION OF THE CORPUS LUTEUM

A further consideration is that up to now we have agreed with Ogino-Knaus that between ovulation and the end of the cycle there is an interval of 16 days at most, *and of 12 days at least*, which corresponds to the duration of the corpus luteum.

Now, although it is true that the corpus luteum cannot last longer than 16 days, *there is nothing to prevent it being shorter than 12 days.* For this it is sufficient that the hormonal secretion of the corpus luteum should dry up prematurely (e.g. from insufficient functioning of the gland). According to the mechanism with which we are now familiar, menstruation will start within the limiting period of 12 days.

It is obvious that the possibility of a shorter corpus luteum phase will entirely upset the Ogino calculation. One can then no longer fix the end of the period of abstention, which is calculated on the supposition that the corpus luteum will last for 12 days at least.

Although the abbreviated duration of the corpus luteum is less common than delay in ovulation, it adds to the uncertainty in determining the end of the period of abstinence which the latter eventuality had already produced.

CONCLUSION

To sum up this critical consideration, it would appear that the method of Ogino-Knaus depends upon two hypothetical calculations:

The first, relating to the first sterile (or "safe") period, may be regarded as reliable and as offering sufficient security: it should be used.

The second, on the other hand, *which is concerned with the end of the period of abstention, offers no security.* One can never be sure then that the resumption of intercourse on the date theoretically allowed by the method can be followed with impunity, *and this alone condemns it.*

If again it be emphasized that the disturbances which may upset calculations, especially delay in ovulation, can happen in the best regulated and normal cycle, it will be clear that the Ogino-Knaus method does not offer sufficient security, even in the most favourable cases where there are regular cycles of normal length.

Does this mean that we must admit defeat, and that women must remain slaves, so to speak, to physiological imperatives which cause the female organism to be liable to a constant recurrence of pregnancy?

We shall see that this is far from being the case, and that there is a way out of this servitude. It is as though Nature, while making sure of the perpetuation of the species, had taken care at the same time to safeguard the liberty of the individual.[1] The way this is done is through the study of the temperature in the course of the menstrual cycle, and upon this is based the method which we will now consider.

[1] We may note in this respect that in women, as we have seen, ovulation simply depends on the degree of maturation of the ovum, without any reference to sexual relations. In this way they differ from most animal species, in which coitus is closely linked with procreation; either because the capacity for coitus is only viable when the female is in a state of fertilizability (in rut or "heat"), or else because coitus itself sets off ovulation, as in the female rabbit (a particularly prolific animal, as is well known).

It would appear, then, that while Nature has arranged matters in the female organism so as to increase the species, she has not made procreation the only goal of sexual relations.

4

THE TEMPERATURE METHOD

LET us consider the temperature curve shown in Fig. 7. It is that of a young woman with normal menstrual periods who has noted her temperature on waking throughout her menstrual cycle.

At first sight this curve looks irregular, festooned with little spikes in a haphazard way, so that one could regard it, maliciously, as an expression of the female character: capricious and wayward!

All the same, this is merely a surface appearance: if we look at the general line of the curve, ignoring the "embroideries", we can see that at the beginning of the cycle the temperature does not go beyond a certain level, which in this case is below 37°C. (98·4°F.). Then, at a given moment, the curve rises progressively to a higher level which is now round 37°C. or a little above, *and remains at this level* until just before the onset of menstruation, when it descends again to its former level.

Let us turn now to the lower curve in Fig. 7, which is that of the menopausal woman. This also shows slight irregularities, but the general line of the curve remains always at the same level; which is the opposite of the one we have just been considering.

THE SIGNIFICANCE OF THESE FACTS

When, as in the menopausal woman, there is no ovarian activity, there will be no rise in the temperature. From this we deduce that the presence of a "thermal plateau" before menstruation is indicative of ovarian activity.

More precisely, we now know that *this pre-menstrual rise of temperature is due to the secretion of the corpus luteum.*

Following the work of Van de Velde in Holland, Rubenstein and Zuck in the U.S.A., and of Palmer in France, it has been scientifically demonstrated that this hormonal secretion has the power to raise temperature.[1]

It follows from this that the thermal curve will run parallel with the hormonal secretion of the corpus

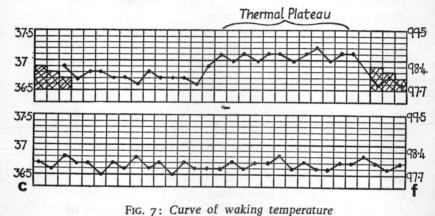

FIG. 7: *Curve of waking temperature*
Above : temperature curve of menstruating woman.
Below : temperature curve of menopausal woman.

luteum, as with the latter the temperature rises by a few tenths of a degree from the moment of ovulation, to reach a higher level which is maintained as long as the hormone secretion of the corpus luteum is continued. When at the end of the cycle the hormone

---

[1] We may recall the fact that in the human species, temperature is regulated with extreme precision by those centres in the nervous system which are termed "heat-regulating centres". These centres, which work just like a thermostat, are concerned with keeping the temperature of the body at a constant level.

secretion dries up, the temperature falls to its original level at the same time as the reappearance of menstruation (Fig. 8).

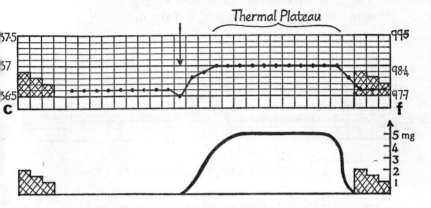

Fig. 8 : *Temperature curve and hormonal curve of the corpus luteum (schematic)*

Above : the temperature curve during the cycle.

Below : the curve of hormonal secretion of corpus luteum during the same cycle (in milligrammes for the 24 hours). The arrow indicates time of ovulation.

LOCALIZATION OF OVULATION ON THE CURVE

Since the temperature rises from the moment of ovulation, the latter will be sited on the curve *just before the rise* in temperature, *at the last dot of low temperature* (Fig. 9, at the arrow).

Experience has shown, however, that ovulation *can also occur at the rise of the curve*, though much more rarely (Fig. 9, hatched zone), and, more precisely, at the beginning of the rise, especially when this occurs gradually.[1]

---

[1] The explanation of this phenomenon is outside the scope of this book. We need merely note that ovulation can vary slightly in relation to the beginning of the rise in temperature.

On the other hand it is an established fact that *ovulation cannot occur later, on the thermal plateau* (this is understandable if it is kept in mind that this plateau is the faithful companion of the corpus luteum, which can form only after discharge of the ovum).

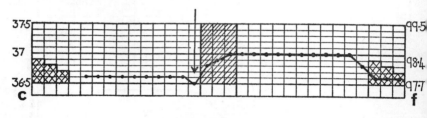

FIG. 9: *Localization of ovulation on the curve*

The arrow indicates the point at which ovulation normally occurs, at the end of the period of low temperature.

Ovulation may, however, equally well occur at the rise of the curve (hatched zone).

PRINCIPLE OF THE THERMAL METHOD

It follows, then, from these facts that *once the temperature has risen, and become stabilized at the level of the thermal plateau, one can be sure that ovulation is already over* and consequently that intercourse can never prove fertile.

The temperature curve has made it possible to solve the difficult problem which was set by the incalculable possibility of delayed ovulation: if ovulation is in fact delayed, the rise in temperature which follows it will also be delayed, as will the plateau following. Therefore by avoiding intercourse until the plateau is established *there is complete assurance against the risk of a delayed ovulation*, a risk which was considerable in the Ogino-Knaus method.

Instead of a theoretical weighing up of probabilities,

the thermal curve method provides, in every individual case, the certitude that ovulation has actually occurred and that there is therefore no risk of pregnancy.

POST-OVULATION SAFE PERIOD

Since the safe period is established when the temperature reaches the ceiling of the thermal plateau, it is incumbent to know when this has been reached; for this it must be confirmed that *the temperature has risen, and has become stabilized* at a level higher than the initial.

One cannot, however, be sure that it *is stabilized* until it has remained at the same level for at least three days in succession; *it is only towards the third or fourth day of the thermal plateau, therefore, that one can be sure of being really on to the premenstrual thermal plateau.*

At this moment, then, one can be sure that intercourse will not prove fertile. In effect, when it is recognized that the thermal plateau has really started, the corpus luteum has already been in existence for three days at least; ovulation has therefore been passed by three days at least, and the period of survival, which is 24 hours at most, has now undoubtedly finished.

From this moment there is a safe period which can be termed *post-ovulation*, since it occurs after ovulation. As there is only one ovulation per cycle[1] this safe

---

[1] There can only be one ovulation per cycle because the corpus luteum prevents other ova from reaching maturity. So long as the corpus luteum is in being, the way is blocked for all other ova, as a train blocks the line behind it when passing certain signals. On the other hand, it is possible for two ova to reach maturity, though rarely, at the same time, and to be fertilized by different sperms : this is what happens in the case of "dissimilar" twins. "Identical" twins correspond to one ovum, fertilized by one sperm, which has subsequently divided.

period continues until the end of the cycle, that is until the onset of fresh menstruation (Fig. 10).

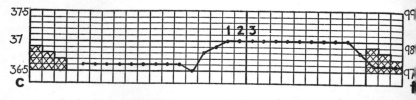

FIG. 10: *Post-ovulation safe period*

This safe period commences on the 3rd day of the thermal plateau and continues until the onset of the next menstruation.

THE INITIAL STERILE PERIOD

At the beginning of the cycle, before the ovum has been released, intercourse cannot be fertile; there is therefore another sterile (safe) period from the beginning of the cycle until ovulation occurs.

Unfortunately the thermal curve does not make it possible to determine the length of this period, because in following the temperature in the course of the cycle, it obviously cannot be known that it is going to rise a few days later.

But, from the fact that the corpus luteum has a maximum life of 16 days, one can be certain that ovulation cannot take place sooner than 16 days before the end of the cycle. If one takes away two days to allow for the possible survival of the sperms, and another day for protection, that is a total of 19 days, then the days which remain at the beginning of the cycle are sterile. In other words, we come back to the calculation of Ogino with regard to the first sterile period: which we recognized as being reliable. We shall then make use of it, therefore, to calculate the first sterile period, the length of which is obtained by taking 19 days from the cycle which has been found to be the shortest hitherto.

Thus, if the shortest cycle has lasted for 26 days, we have a safe period of 26 − 19, i.e. 7, days at the beginning of the cycle.

Conclusion: The General Line to be Followed

To sum up, the length of the initial safe period, which cannot be foretold from the temperature, can be properly determined from the Ogino calculation, which affords sufficient security in this respect. On the other hand, the end of the period of abstention, for which the Ogino calculation is of no value, can be determined through the temperature curve with all the degree of security required.

From these findings we deduce the general line to be followed by those wishing to practise period abstention (Fig. 11).

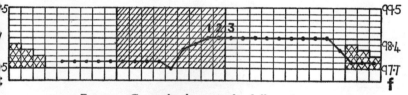

FIG. 11 : *General scheme to be followed*

After making use of the days available at the beginning of the cycle, which as we have seen are calculated from the shortest cycle previously noted, abstention is practised until the temperature has risen and become stabilized at the top level for at least three days (hatching on diagram).

1. *A certain number of days of sterility are available at the beginning of the cycle.* The length of this first safe period depends on the shortest cycle previously noted, and is calculated by subtracting 19 days from the length of the cycle.

2. Following this, the temperature is carefully noted and *abstention practised so long as the temperature remains low*, i.e. at the initial level.

3. Intercourse is not resumed until the temperature has *risen* and *maintained its high level for at least three days.*

In short, after using the days which are available at the beginning of the cycle, it is simply a case of waiting for the appearance of the "thermal plateau". Such is the very simple rule which results from using the temperature method.

5

KNOWLEDGE OF THE CYCLE BY MEANS OF THE TEMPERATURE CURVE

THE interest of the temperature curve does not only consist in the fact that it provides a sure and simple method of estimating the fertile and infertile parts of the cycle. It gives us most valuable and precise knowledge as to the menstrual cycle itself.

We will see how it is possible, by this simple means, for any woman who so desires to acquire a knowledge of her menstrual cycle, the interest of which—on the intellectual or psychological point of view, or that of physical hygiene—hardly needs stressing.

TEMPERATURE CURVE AND VARIATIONS OF CYCLE

If we can talk of the "inconstant female" we can afford to be indulgent towards her—when we consider the infinite variations of the menstrual cycle: how it varies from one woman to another, and often in the same woman from one cycle to another.

To say that a cycle has lasted 28, 35, or 22 days gives us no information whatever as to the nature or the reasons for this variation; whereas the temperature curve is going to yield very exact information on this point.

In order to understand the matter, we must recall the structure of the cycle: how the *follicular phase*, which terminates in ovulation, lasts normally for 14 days, but may be shorter or longer than this period, when follicular maturation is disturbed. These variations in the date of ovulation obviously bring about corresponding variations in the length of the cycle, which is shortened

31

when ovulation is advanced, and lengthened when ovulation is retarded.

Coming now to the *luteal phase*, of which the duration is usually 14 days, we know that it cannot be prolonged for longer than 16 days, but, on the other hand, that it can be shorter than its average length, if for any reason the hormone secretion of the corpus luteum is prematurely stopped. In such a case, obviously, the cycle will be correspondingly shorter.

These various changes in the menstrual cycle can combine, either to increase their joint effects, or to compensate each other.[1]

Add to this the fact that these changes may happen habitually or accidentally, and one can realize the infinite variety of menstrual cycles, which appear to have no rhyme or reason.

But it must be noted that in every case the temperature curve gives us both the date of ovulation and the duration of the corpus luteum, that is to say, the two basic elements the variations of which bring about those of the menstrual cycle.

Thanks, then, to the temperature curve, it is always possible to recognize what the particular cycle consists of, to follow its variations, and to explain its mechanism. *The thermal curve, like Ariadne's thread, will always enable you to find your way through the labyrinth of the cycles.*

THE ANOVULAR CYCLE

Now here is a paradoxical situation: we have seen how the menstrual cycle revolves entirely round ovula-

---

[1] Thus, ovulation on the 20th day, followed by a corpus luteum of 8 days, gives a cycle of (20 + 8), i.e. 28 days, which, far from being normal, shows a double anomaly, namely retardation of ovulation, and shortening of the duration of the corpus luteum.

tion, which is in fact its *raison d'être*. But, however strange at first sight, there may be a menstrual cycle without ovulation.

This type of cycle, known as "anovular", is found in cases of wrong functioning of the glands; either at the beginning of sexual life, when the mechanism of ovulation is not yet established, or at the end of sexual life, when the ageing ovary no longer has the capacity to assure ovulation at each cycle.

From what we know as to the mechanism of menstruation, it will seem strange that a cycle with no ovulation, hence with no corpus luteum, can still produce menstruation. In fact, menstruation is then produced by the intervention of another ovarian hormone which we have purposely not mentioned as yet. This hormone, manufactured by the follicle itself, hence named "follicular", has the task of preparing the uterine mucous lining for the action of the corpus luteum hormone. Even in the absence of the latter, however, it can bring about menstruation through an analogous mechanism. This "folliculine', however, is not subject to any time sequence, and its length may be anything. From this it follows that the cycle can exhibit the most fantastic variations, which are characteristic of the period preceding the real menopause.

The absence of ovulation is therefore yet another cause for variations in the cycle. Moreover, the absence of ovulation may be habitual or accidental: anovular alternating with ovular cycles so that there may be a still greater variety in menstrual cycles.

But here again the temperature curve comes to our aid by providing easy recognition of an "anovular" cycle: if there is no corpus luteum there will be no corresponding hormonal secretion and consequently no rise in temperature. The temperature will therefore remain at the same level at which it started, during the whole of the menstrual cycle, and the curve becomes a flat one, like that of the menopause (Fig. 12).

Thus, under all circumstances, even when the vagaries of the cycle are tied up with the absence of ovulation, the temperature curve gives us the explanation.

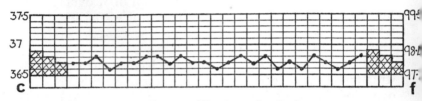

FIG. 12: *The Anovular Cycle*

The temperature remains at the same level throughout the cycle.

MEDICAL KNOWLEDGE OF THE CYCLE

The knowledge of the cycle which is given by the temperature curve is, as may be supposed, of the utmost value to the physician himself.

The thermal curve will give him information, far more readily than any long description, about the menstrual cycle: telling him whether there is ovulation or not, what is its place in the cycle, and what the duration of the corpus luteum; it is obvious how important this information can be.

These indications are of particular value when menstruation is irregular, or accompanied by haemorrhages, so that the patient is no longer able to distinguish the one from the other. The temperature curve provides an easy way to find the solution: the patient can recognize normal menstruation by the fact that it is preceded by the thermal plateau. Conversely, *every bleeding which does not coincide with the fall in temperature should be considered abnormal* and requiring advice from the doctor.

Thus, thanks to the thermal curve, it is possible to

discover in good time those conditions which it might not be possible to cure if treatment is left too late.

Many women, with the idea of helping the doctor's diagnosis, make detailed notes of their symptoms. But the doctor cannot gain much information from these facts, however meticulously noted down, if he does not know at what particular moment of the cycle these symptoms became manifest.

Thus, in order to decide whether a given symptom, for example a severe migraine, has some connection with an endocrine disorder or not, it is of importance to know whether it comes on always at the same time within the cycle, e.g. at the time of ovulation or at the premenstrual period.

The temperature curve, and only this, enables one to place the symptoms in relation to the different phases of the cycle: it is therefore a fundamental factor in diagnosis.

The temperature curve is also indispensable when complementary investigations are considered necessary to solve a diagnostic problem.

For example, if it is desired to study the function of the corpus luteum, it is obviously necessary to carry out the required investigations (such as collecting a specimen of urine) when there is a corpus luteum present. This, as we have seen, can vary the time of its appearance in the cycle. In collecting a specimen on a fixed date, e.g. the 21st day of the cycle, when there ought in theory to be a corpus luteum, one cannot be sure of finding one in fact. On the other hand, nothing is easier with the thermal curve, which allows us to follow the traces of the corpus luteum, thanks to the thermal plateau. With a specimen of urine collected at the time of this plateau, one is sure of lighting upon the corpus luteum.

D

If the patient herself knows at what precise moment this analysis can be effectively carried out, she can be of great help to her physician; with consequent benefit to herself.

It is important to note that *if the temperature curve is not observed, it is not possible to interpret the results of an endocrine analysis in the woman*: in point of fact, the values of the different endocrine secretions are not the same at different parts of the cycle. Without the temperature curve, it is not possible to establish the exact moment of the cycle and consequently what the values were which should be found at the time. Failure to observe the temperature renders it impossible for the doctor to make use of the information thus gathered, often with some trouble, and thus one may miss the benefits of these modern methods of diagnosis.

But the temperature curve is not only of service in endocrinological diagnosis; it is of equal importance in treatment and clinical supervision.

Certain drugs have to be given at specified moments in the cycle, and the temperature curve is then able to guide the treatment by indicating the favourable moment. It also provides control of the efficiency of treatment when, for example, it is a question of re-establishing a disturbance of the luteal function: the reappearance of the normal thermal plateau will then indicate the success of the treatment. Again, thanks to the information which one can provide for the doctor, it makes it possible for him to supervise his patient from a distance, which is of advantage in case of absence.[1]

This bird's-eye view gives some idea of the incomparable services which the temperature curve can render in

[1] See p. 67: cyclo-thermic chart.

the diagnosis and treatment of menstrual troubles. So true is this that it is impossible to care adequately for a woman with menstrual troubles without the help of the temperature curve, which is now seen to be an indispensable aid to the doctor.[1] In observing her temperature, a woman will have the satisfaction not only of controlling her sexual life and being conscious of it, but will also contribute in no small measure towards maintaining her health.

[1] Cf. S. Geller: *La courbe thermique, guide du Praticien en Endocrinologie feminine*, Masson, Paris, 1961.

6

THE TEMPERATURE CURVE
AND PREGNANCY

THE temperature curve, so valuable during the menstrual cycle, is no less so in time of pregnancy, which is, as we have seen, the natural end and purpose of the menstrual cycle, through which the woman realizes her real biological destiny: which is to transmit new life.

USE OF THE TEMPERATURE CURVE WITH A VIEW TO PREGNANCY

The temperature curve is not only concerned with periodic abstinence, but is also a means of achieving a desired pregnancy.

By establishing the moment in the cycle when ovulation occurs, the thermal curve indicates the time of maximum concentration when the chances of fertility are at their greatest. It is therefore a useful aid to those couples whose fertility is doubtful, and no gynaecologist today would ignore it.

It is equally of interest when it is desirable to choose the date of the birth; for example in order to avoid the child being born at the time of great heat, when it may be exposed to the danger of digestive troubles.

We might add that it is not a matter of indifference, as stressed by Knaus,[1] that at the time of conception the reproductive cells should not be weakened by a transient physical disorder in the parents, and also that conception should take place at the time when the reproductive cells are at the maximum of their capacity for fertility. By thus permitting couples who desire to

[1] H. Knaus, *Fécondité périodique et procréation volontaire.*

choose the date of conception, making allowance for their state of health, and enabling them to fix the time of ovulation with greater accuracy, the temperature curve serves their legitimate desire to conceive their children under the most favourable conditions.

WHAT HAPPENS IN THE TIME OF PREGNANCY

The sperm, by fertilizing the ovum, has, in a sense, saved it from perishing. The egg which results from this encounter will now survive and become implanted in the uterine mucosa which, carefully prepared by the corpus luteum, will now offer it the best conditions for developing.

At the end of a few days, this tiny egg has already acquired sufficient vitality to produce a new hormone which will stimulate the corpus luteum at the very moment when the latter would have run its course and ceased to secrete.

Thanks to this admirable arrangement, the secretion of the corpus luteum, instead of drying up, will go on and will continue to accumulate the precious nutritive substances in the uterine mucosa, which are indispensable for the life of the egg. The uterine mucosa will thus continue to proliferate, and the expected menstruation will not come on: this being the first sign of pregnancy, as everyone knows.

THE TEMPERATURE AT THE BEGINNING OF PREGNANCY

Since, as we have just seen, the corpus luteum continues to secrete in pregnancy, the thermal plateau, its inseparable companion, will continue well beyond the limited period of 16 days which was characteristic of the corpus luteum of the cycle (Fig. 13).

From this it is possible to deduce an extremely simple rule, within everyone's reach, in order to recognize pregnancy: if menstruation is delayed, and if having observed the temperature from the beginning of the cycle it is noted that *it has risen* to its upper level *and has maintained this level for longer than* 16 *days*, it is likely that pregnancy has started.[1]

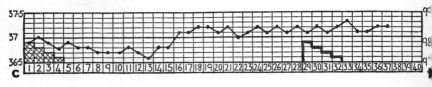

FIG. 13 : *The temperature in a case of pregnancy*

In the case of pregnancy the expected menses do not happen and the temperature is maintained at the high level.

Conversely, *even though the menses are late in appearing, pregnancy is not likely if the temperature remains at the same level as at the beginning of the cycle*: if the temperature has not risen this means indeed that there has been no ovulation and therefore no pregnancy.[2]

FURTHER EVOLUTION OF THE TEMPERATURE

In the case of pregnancy, the thermal plateau will remain the same until about the 4th month of gestation, at which point the temperature will come down once more to its level at the beginning of the cycle.

At this time the corpus luteum of pregnancy, which was concerned simply with the start of the pregnancy, will now be replaced by a new and more potent endocrine gland, namely the placenta, which has been form-

[1] However, as it is not always easy to estimate within one day or two the exact beginning of the thermal plateau, it is advisable to wait about 20 days to be sure.

[2] It may be the case either of a cycle without ovulation, or of a cycle in which it has been retarded, in which case it may still be produced. It will be necessary to envisage this latter possibility if pregnancy is not desired.

ing at the site where the egg has become implanted in the uterine mucous membrane. The hormones of the placenta will now allow of the general development of pregnancy, but will not influence the temperature as did the hormone secretion of the corpus luteum; this is why, at this point, when the corpus luteum has ceased to be active, the temperature falls to its initial level,[1] where it will remain until the delivery.

The Temperature Curve and the Stage of Pregnancy

When a woman seeks a consultation about her pregnancy, the first question the doctor will put will be: "What was the date of your last period?" It is indeed from the date of the last period that the stage of pregnancy is usually calculated, and this is a fundamental factor in estimating the normality of the pregnancy.

It may be that there is some hesitation over the exact date of the last period, especially if menstruation has been irregular, or if, what not unusually happens, there has been slight bleeding with the first missed period.

Moreover, even if the date of the last period is accurately known, the exact stage of the pregnancy is not thereby determined with certainty, because pregnancy does not actually start with the last period but with fertilization, that is to say, at the time when ovulation has taken place in the fertile cycle. As ovulation may have taken place at any moment in this cycle, and especially with some delay, knowing the date of the last period does not give information about the *exact* stage of pregnancy.

On the other hand, the temperature curve makes it possible to establish the date of ovulation in the fertile cycle as in other cycles. It will therefore fix with

[1] This explanation is only approximative. The true one would be beyond the scope of this book.

accuracy the true beginning and exact stage of the pregnancy and thus provide valuable information for its general supervision. It cannot therefore be too strongly urged that women who desire to go through pregnancy under the best possible conditions should take note of their temperature during the fertile cycle.

THE CONFINEMENT

The hormone secretion of the placenta continues and increases right through pregnancy, and will only cease when the development of the foetus is complete. Just as, at the end of the cycle, the fall in the secretion of the corpus luteum meant the reappearance of menstruation, so the fall in the amount of this hormone at the end of pregnancy brings about the process which initiates delivery.

THE TEMPERATURE CURVE AND MISCARRIAGE

If the fall in hormone secretion occurs before the end of pregnancy, it will be clear that this will bring about the detachment of the foetus in the same manner, and consequently produce a miscarriage or a premature delivery. In fact nowadays hormonal deficiency is considered to be one of the most likely causes of miscarriage, and particularly of frequent miscarriages occurring in successive pregnancies.

In these cases the fall in hormonal secretion happens gradually as a rule. It is therefore possible to discover this by hormone analysis, and to correct it by appropriate treatment before it is too late.

But this deficiency is often produced from the beginning of pregnancy,[1] and in order to avoid miscarriage it is essential to carry out hormone analysis from the very beginning of pregnancy. The temperature curve

[1] From the fact that the corpus luteum stops its secretion before the placenta begins to function.

will then show its great usefulness by enabling pregnancy to be recognized as present from the very first days "missed". Thanks to this, it is now possible to carry out hormone analysis from the very beginning of pregnancy, and thus to establish the best condition for the preventive treatment of miscarriages.

THE TEMPERATURE CURVE AND THE RETURN OF MENSTRUATION

After confinement (as indeed after miscarriage), a new cycle starts which will end with the resumption of menstruation which will generally occur about six weeks after the confinement.

This cycle, which finishes on the resumption of menstruation, is rather special, because the mechanism of ovular maturation, which has been blocked all through pregnancy, takes a certain time to resume its normal function.

Generally speaking, this cycle does not involve ovulation, hence pregnancy, and the temperature will remain at its basal level until the return of menstruation.

But this is not always the case; it may happen that the cycle produces ovulation, and a corpus luteum. In this case, after a varying interval, the temperature is seen to rise and the thermal plateau which heralds the resumption of menstruation will be noted. Obviously in such a case pregnancy is a possibility. But as one cannot tell in advance if the temperature is about to rise or to stay at its low level, one cannot possibly be sure that intercourse before the return of menstruation may not be followed by pregnancy.

As this is not desirable at that time, for obvious reasons, *prudence is necessary when resuming intercourse after a confinement.*

The safest course indeed would be to imitate the Touaregs, whose custom it is that the wife should be separated from the husband until the return of menstruation.

The temperature curve, however, permits of a less radical solution: *it suffices to abstain so long as the temperature remains low*. Only the reappearance of the thermal plateau and its persistence for three days can guarantee that intercourse will not result in pregnancy.

THE TEMPERATURE CURVE AND DELAY IN THE RETURN OF MENSTRUATION

However, the reappearance of the menses may be delayed, particularly if the woman is breast-feeding.

In such a case, if intercourse has taken place one may wonder whether another pregnancy is on the way.

This problem will be easily solved if the temperature has been taken regularly since the confinement: if the temperature is all the time at its low level, one may be sure that it is not a pregnancy, but a simple delay in the return of menstruation.[1]

If, on the other hand, the temperature has been seen to rise and to remain at the high level for more than 20 days, one may well conclude that it is most likely a case of pregnancy.[2]

Thus the temperature, which is a faithful reflection of the corpus luteum in the cycle, equally faithfully reflects the activity of the corpus luteum of pregnancy, and also, when this exists, the corpus luteum preceding the return of the menses which announce the resumption of the cyclic sexual life.

[1] In this case it is best to ask the doctor to procure the return of the menses, which is usually an easy matter.

[2] If the temperature has risen, and has remained at the higher level for less than 16 days, it may still indicate the thermal plateau preceding the return of menses. It will then suffice to wait a few more days to settle the matter.

7

FROM PUBERTY TO THE MENOPAUSE

To conclude this brief account of the uses of the temperature, we can now consider the thermal curve in a kind of panoramic view of sexual life, from puberty to the menopause.

PUBERTY

Puberty in the young girl is marked officially by the appearance of menstruation. In fact, however, this first menstrual period is but the concluding phase of a long continued underground process, through which, as though by some mysterious alchemy, the young girl gradually takes shape. The breasts develop, the pelvic cavity widens, the hips get broader—where, some day, a new life will appear and be sheltered. Even in the psychic sphere, with the appearance of modesty, coquetry, and the delicate awakening of the senses, there is a process of transformation preparing the organism of the young girl for her feminine role.

The ground being thus prepared by this slow hormonal development, one day a follicle, like an opening bud, reaches maturity and opens to shed the first ovum. Within this now open bud the first corpus luteum will blossom, expand and then fade; its disappearance being followed by the first menstrual period: showing forth the complete metamorphosis of the chrysalis. The first cycle will be followed by another, and so on. . . .

It may happen, however, that the first menstrual period, and the first few that will follow, will not involve the formation of a corpus luteum, as indicated by the thermal curve, which in this case will remain flat.

Often, however, everything is soon in order, as shown by the thermal curve, which now assumes its normal appearance.

But sometimes things go wrong, and the cycle, which cannot proceed for long without the corpus luteum, becomes really disturbed: long intervals without menstruation alternating with very profuse and even haemorrhagic periods.

The temperature curve in such cases is of the utmost use, rendering it possible in many cases to discover the cause of the trouble, namely the absence of the corpus luteum, and to take necessary therapeutic measures.

Thus, from the beginnings of sexual life, the temperature curve proves its usefulness by making it possible to control the physiological functions of puberty, and discover possible abnormalities. Mothers who are concerned for the good health of their daughters would be well advised to get them into the habit of taking their temperature from the beginning of menstruation.

Cyclic Sexual Life

Either from the beginning after the first menstrual period, or after some initial fumbling, ovarian function will assume its normal cyclic rhythm. Hereafter the menstrual cycles will succeed each other regularly, with the two phases with which we are now familiar, based upon the process of ovulation. Every woman will have a particular type of cycle which can be recognized by means of the temperature curve.

All the same, even if this is regular and normal, it may be subject to accidental modifications, of which the most important would be the possible delay in ovulation. This eventuality, where the Ogino-Knaus method proved powerless, does not offer any problem with the thermal curve, which provides automatic assurance against this danger.

But the menstrual cycle can also change and evolve during the course of sexual life. One woman who starts with a cycle of normal length may find this cycle getting longer or shorter; another who has up to now been like clock-work may find some fine day that her cycle is describing fantastic variations; yet another, whose cycle was at first irregular, may see it becoming gradually normal in the latter years of her sex life.

As in the case of accidental variations, the temperature curve can also uncover the evolutionary modifications of the menstrual cycle, which can of course upset the most learned calculations. Thanks to the subtlety of this procedure, which follows the slightest variations in the life of the ovary, it is possible, as we have seen, to recognize the new type of cycle when it makes its appearance, and act accordingly.

PREGNANCY

The slow hormonal development which turns a graceful girl into a young woman perfectly adapted for her feminine role; the hormonal outflow which, like the joyful preparation for a marriage which is continually postponed, untiringly prepares the uterine mucosa at each cycle to receive the fertilized egg; finally, the hormonal impulses which underlie mutual sexual attraction: all of these are tending towards the woman's supreme achievement—pregnancy.

It will not be necessary to refer any further to this topic, which has been discussed at such length, nor to the advantages of the temperature curve in helping to achieve pregnancy. We need only note that the resumption of menstruation closes the circuit of events which are set off by the fertilization of the ovum. Another cycle will follow; the round of cycles which has been temporarily interrupted will be complete once more, and cyclic sexual life resume its course.

THE MENOPAUSE

Sexual life, then, whether or not interrupted by pregnancy, will continue until the ageing ovary is no longer able to regulate the maturation of the ovum; ovulation will then occur only intermittently or irregularly, until it disappears completely.

The cycles then become irregular (either from variation in the time of ovulation, or occasional anovular cycles). Disturbances of varying degree, particularly haemorrhage, may result. Even in the absence of major disturbances, these irregularities may present problems from the fact that some cycles may include ovulation, hence the possibility of pregnancy.

Thanks to the temperature curve, which indicates whether or not there is ovulation, and in the first instance what is its place in the cycle, it is easy to understand these variations, to treat the disturbances which go with them, and to protect oneself against the possibility of a pregnancy, which would be inopportune at such a time of life (see pp. 65 and 66).

In any case the ovarian function, after some false starts which are responsible for the troubles at what is called "the critical age", will cease: this is the menopause properly so called, when the woman, her biological potentialities now resolved, can at last reach the serenity of a life without cycles.[1]

The temperature curve is no longer of use to her, but has proved to be her sure and faithful guide throughout the years of her sexual life.

[1] But also without the beneficent effects of her cyclic hormonal impregnation, hence the symptoms of "defeminization" which can be seen at this time of life. Thanks, however, to synthetic hormones produced by modern pharmacology, it is possible to bring about "artificial cycles" which, with only the illusion of a sexual life, nevertheless furnish the menopausal woman with the beneficial general effects of hormonal impregnation.

PART TWO

PRACTICAL APPLICATIONS OF THE TEMPERATURE METHOD

It now remains to tackle the practical side: here will be found details of what it is necessary to know, in order to reap the advantages of the temperature curve.

HOW IS THE TEMPERATURE
TO BE TAKEN?

THIS question may sound superfluous. Nevertheless it is fundamental: we have to establish variations of temperature within tenths of degrees. In order to get precise information from the temperature curve, it has to be observed under very definite conditions:

1. *The temperature must be taken on waking in the morning, before setting foot to the ground.*

It must be pointed out that the simple act of getting up causes the temperature to rise by several tenths of a degree, which obviously upsets the curve. It must therefore be taken *before rising.*[1]

2. *The temperature must be taken at the same time every day.*

It must be realized that the temperature is not the same at different hours of the day, and that it is higher in the evening than in the morning. If therefore it is desired to compare the figures from one day to another, it is necessary to take the temperature every day *at about the same time.*[2]

3. *The temperature should be taken rectally.*

[1] One may forget and get up. In this case one can go back to bed and still note the temperature, remembering that on that day it has been taken after getting up and may be a little higher. On the other hand if one has got up during the night, the waking temperature is quite valid if one has been back in bed for over an hour.

[2] It may happen that on some days one gets up at a different hour to the usual. In such a case one should remember that the temperature will be a little higher if taken a bit later, and slightly lower if taken a little earlier (the difference being about a tenth of a degree per hour). It is therefore advisable to mark the temperatures taken at unusual times with coloured pencil.

This is because rectal temperature is by far the most precise and accurate. However, oral temperatures, though less reliable, may also be used, if one is very particular about it. But it must be emphasized that it does not provide such a good security.[1]

In résumé:—rectal temperature;
          —taken in the morning before rising;
          —about the same time each day.

These conditions are therefore very simple. But they must be strictly observed in order to get the benefits of the temperature curve.

If these conditions are not adhered to, it is no longer possible to trust to temperature readings. By neglecting them one is exposed to possible bitter disappointment with no one to blame but oneself. *It is better not to take temperature at all than to take it badly.*

HOW TO NOTE THE TEMPERATURE

The observed temperature should be put down *on a suitable graph paper.*

In fact it is not sufficient to note the temperature on a bit of paper; *it is necessary to trace the curve*, which is much more telling than a row of figures.

On the other hand, the characteristics of the curve do not emerge clearly on ordinary charts marked in two-tenths, and errors may occur. A chart especially designed for the temperature of the cycle is indicated. It is therefore proposed that a model chart, which will be found at the end of the book, should be used, which has been designed to show in the clearest manner the characteristics of the curve. Moreover, this chart allows for the noting down, day by day, of all information which is useful for a study of the cycle.

[1] As oral values are slightly lower, it may be necessary in this case to lower the figures of the model chart, p. 75 (for instance enter 36° instead of 36.5°; 36.5° instead of 37°, etc.).

And here is a simple piece of advice: place the temperature chart, together with the thermometer and a pencil, at the bedside; one will then have everything required within reach, and can be sure not to forget. By forming a habit, one need not worry any more. Now for the question in everybody's mind:

FOR HOW LONG MUST THE TEMPERATURE BE TAKEN?

Rest assured: it is not necessary to spend all one's life riveted to the thermometer!

No doubt at first it is as well to note the temperature throughout the cycle, in order to familiarize oneself with the general line of the curve. But quite soon, after a few cycles, the temperature may be taken only from the moment when the first sterile (safe) period has elapsed, and, as soon as the thermal plateau is clearly evident, the thermometer can be abandoned. In other words, *it will only be necessary to note the temperature during the time necessary to recognize the thermal shift*, which implies at most a dozen days per month; which is not asking too much.[1]

It has been said that not many women would submit themselves to this slavery with the necessary patience and conscientiousness; this shows a poor appreciation of what women are capable of. Every gynaecologist knows how much patience they can show if they so desire. How could it be otherwise when it is a question of such fundamental importance as their sexual life? In fact it is just such a habit as is required for the hygiene of every day. It is also a discipline in which a woman vindicates her emancipation. Is not this far more worthy of a being dowered with reason than drugs or gadgets to prevent conception? The satisfaction of

[1] This reduced notation of the temperature usually suffices also for its medical use.

knowing where one stands, of being aware of one's physiological state, of being master of one's fate: these are adequate compensations.

As for those who fear that this practice takes away the poesy of love, we can ask them what becomes of the poesy when this leads to an unwanted pregnancy, becoming in some cases a major catastrophe—when it does not lead to desperate measures, confessed in lamentable terms to us doctors in our consulting rooms?

HOW TO DETERMINE THE INITIAL SAFE PERIOD

WE have seen that in order to calculate the first sterile period, 19 days must be subtracted from the shortest cycle observed during the past year.

1. *It is necessary therefore to start by determining the length of each cycle in the current year.*

Now, it will be recalled that the cycle starts on the first day of menstruation[1] (which is also the first day of the cycle). To calculate the length of each cycle, therefore, every day from the day when menstruation begins (inclusive) until the day (exclusive) when the next menstruation starts (this being the first day of the following cycle) must be counted.

Example: If the menses have started on July 9th, and again on August 6th, all days from July 9th (inclusive) to the 6th August (exclusive) must be counted, which is 28 days.

N.B.: The first safe period cannot be accurately determined unless all dates of the commencement of the menses are known, *without exception*. When one starts to practise the method, this information may be lacking

---

[1] If menses start before retiring to bed, that day counts as the first day of menstruation; if menses start after retiring to bed, the next day counts as the first day.

because one has failed to note the beginning dates of the menses, as one should.

In this case, thanks to the temperature curve, it is always possible to make use of the post-ovulation safe period, for which it is not necessary to know the length of cycles. This is indeed one of the many advantages of the thermal method over the Ogino-Knaus.

2. After this, take *the shortest of the cycles and subtract 19 days*; the number of days remaining represent the duration of the first sterile (safe) period.

Example: If it is found that the shortest cycle is one of 26 days, there will be (26 − 19) i.e. 7 days at one's disposal at the beginning of the cycle.

N.B.: The sterile period thus calculated begins on the first day of the cycle, i.e. the first day of the menses, which are consequently included within this period. From this it follows that the menses are generally "safe". However, if the menses are prolonged, the last days may outlast the safe period: thus in the case where the menses last 8 days, and the calculation has given an initial period of 7 days only, the last day of the menses would not be safe.

APPRECIATION OF THE THERMAL SHIFT

Whether it is a case of regulating births or of its medical applications, the essence of the thermal curve consists in knowing at what point the temperature has passed from its low level to the level of the thermal plateau; in other words that it has "shifted".

It must first be emphasized that the absolute value of the temperature has no importance as such. In the example given at the beginning of the book, corresponding to the usual rule, the curve started well below 37°C., and the thermal plateau reached a ceiling round

37°C. But the curve may be found to be displaced in its entirety either towards higher or lower temperatures (Fig. 14). *The level at which the curve will start may therefore be very variable*, and this even in the same woman, from one cycle to another. *The* DIFFERENCE IN THE LEVEL *as between the two parts of the curve is all that counts*, and the whole problem lies in being able to appreciate that the temperature has really passed on to its higher level.

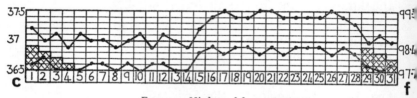

FIG. 14: *High and low curves*

For this it is necessary to establish that the temperature *has risen* in relation to its level at the start, then that *it has become stablized at its higher level*, which implies, as we have seen, that *the temperature remains at this higher level for at least three days*.

Sometimes the rise is quick, in a day or two, and the beginning of the thermal plateau is rectilinear. This type of rise, like a steep bank (Fig. 15A), shows very clearly the difference of levels, and leaves no doubt about the beginning of the thermal plateau, which is easy to recognize from the third day.

Often, however, the rise is gradual, in three or four days, but the beginning of the plateau remains rectilinear and is recognized quickly (Fig. 15 B).

The rise may even take place in a more gradual manner, in 4 or 6 days for example, in "steps" or else in "saw teeth" (Figs. 15 C and D). There is nothing abnormal about these fashions, but it is as well to examine them more closely, because it may at times be a difficult

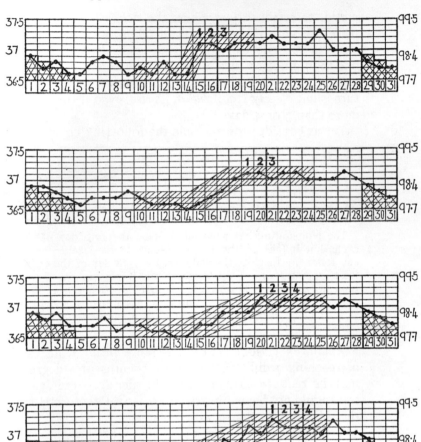

FIG. 15: Aspects of the thermal shift

matter to establish just where the rise finishes and the plateau begins; there is a risk of taking what is only a stage in the rise for the plateau itself. In these cases one should not be in a hurry to draw conclusions, and it is best to *continue to abstain so long as the temperature is not clearly stabilized in its rise,* even if this takes more than 3 or 4 days.

Let us consider for example the following curve.[1]

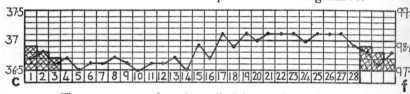

The temperature has risen all right on the 17th day of the cycle, but it falls on the following day, to rise again on the day following that. At this date, i.e. the 19th day of the cycle, the temperature is not yet stabilized and it is necessary to continue to abstain. It is only on the 21st day that one is in a position to know that the temperature is properly stabilized at its higher level, and that one is in a position to resume intercourse.

Again, exceptionally, the difference in level, instead of reaching a difference of 4- or 5-tenths of a degree, *may be reduced to 2- or 3-tenths merely.* Here again one should not be in a hurry to resume intercourse from the third day of the supposed plateau.

It is better to wait for a sufficient length of time to be able to judge that, however slight the difference in levels, there is, notwithstanding, a real difference of level between the two parts of the curve.

Thus, in the curve on p. 59, the temperature has risen on the 15th day and remains on the plateau the follow-

[1] It is advisable to look at this curve, and others, by means of a frame which can be moved from left to right, in order to follow the progress of the curve from day to day, as it shows itself in practice when one follows the temperature through the cycle.

ing days; but the difference is only one of 2-tenths. One should therefore not be in a hurry to resume intercourse from the 3rd day of the thermal plateau, which is in this case the 17th day of the cycle. Nevertheless, it is noted that on the following day and the day after, the temperature is still on the higher level. Despite the slight difference, it can be seen that it was a thermal plateau, and that it is safe to resume intercourse.

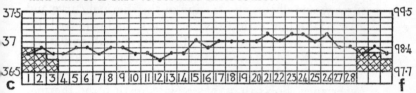

We have purposely dwelt at some length on the difficulties which may be met with in reading the thermal shift, but this is no cause for alarm, and there is no need to suppose that this discussion usually raises insuperable difficulties. In actual fact a few months' practice renders one familiar with the problem, and one is surprised to find how *the curve speaks for itself.* It is simply a matter of habit; an education of the eye which comes from reading the curves and which anyone can master. In fact, apart from a few conditions which are frankly abnormal and belong to the doctor,[1] the reading of the curve poses few problems, and any woman, with a little goodwill and attention, can achieve it.

[1] It may happen indeed that the thermal curve is so irregular that it is not possible to recognize the thermal plateau. But luckily such cases are very rare; excepting always those cases where the temperature has been incorrectly taken (in fact a number of curves which appear abnormal or puzzling are due to the fact that the conditions for taking the temperature properly have not been kept to: it has been taken after rising, at different times, etc.). For the most part these rare cases are due to glandular disorders which are in the province of the doctor. Therefore if there is any difficulty about reading the thermal curve, it should be shown to the doctor.

FALSE RISES

(ABNORMAL TEMPERATURES)

But, you may object, if I am suffering from a cold, influenza, sore throat, or any infectious illness, my temperature will rise; will I not confuse this fever with the rise of temperature which follows ovulation?

One might indeed fear that these abnormal temperatures would distort the tracing of the thermal curve and give a false impression that ovulation had occurred. By resuming intercourse after this pretended ovulation, there might be a danger of striking the real ovulation.

Actually, the danger is far less than one might think; experience shows that these fevers disturb the thermal curve far less than one might suppose, and its accuracy is quite surprising. Besides, it is generally quite easy to unmask these false rises in temperature.

To start with, a rise of temperature happening before the expected date should arouse suspicion.

Secondly, the rise in temperature attributable to the abnormal fevers is usually much greater than that of the thermal shift of ovulation, which is rarely greater than 5-tenths of a degree. Therefore one must be on guard, *a priori*, against greater rises.

Finally, and above all, these extra rises are followed by an irregular fall, and not by a persistent thermal plateau such as is found after ovulation. For protection, therefore, it is enough *to make sure that the suspect rise is really followed by a sustained thermal plateau,*[1] *and to wait sufficiently long to make sure that the plateau is well established.*

---

[1] One should not yield to a common impulse and stop taking the temperature because one is feverish. On the contrary, it is by continuing to take it that it will become evident whether this temperature is or is not followed by a sustained thermal plateau.

Thus in the following curve:

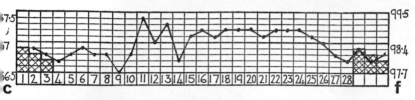

The temperature starts to rise from the 10th day, which is already suspicious. The following day it rises by five points, and this unaccustomed rise is equally suspect. On the days following, the temperature, instead of getting stabilized, comes down irregularly. Abstention is, therefore, still necessary. On the other hand, as from the 19th day, it is evident that the temperature has become stable at a level well above the initial one, and shows an unmistakable plateau. From now on intercourse can be resumed.

Moreover, the symptoms of the illness in question (cold, sore throat, influenza) will have been noticed, so it will be obvious that these abnormal temperatures do not involve any serious risk, and that familiarity with one's own curve will make it easy to recognize their origin.

USE OF THE TEMPERATURE
ACCORDING TO THE CYCLE

SHORT CYCLE.—The shorter the cycle, the more the initial safe period is reduced. Thus, if the shortest cycle is one of only 21 days, the initial period is reduced to (21 − 19), i.e. 2 days.

With short cycles, the calculation may lead to a fairly considerable reduction in the initial sterile period.

If the cycle is very short, it may even result in suppressing this initial safe period altogether. Nevertheless, whatever the situation may be, the thermal curve always makes it possible to keep the post-ovulation safe period, which can be used in any circumstance. Intercourse will then be restricted to the post-ovulation period, after the rise in temperature (Fig. 16).

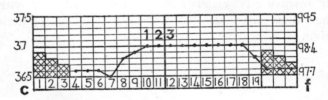

FIG. 16 : *Short Cycle* (schematic)

19-day cycle. The initial period is suppressed. The post-ovulation period is still available.

It should also be noted that, thanks to the thermal curve, it is possible to improve the situation with regard to these short cycles, and to recover some part of the initial period. But this requires rather a subtle use of the curve, presupposing some practice with the method.

For those who are interested, an explanation is given in the Appendix at the end of the book (cf. pp. 76-77).

Long Cycle.—It is considered that a cycle is long when it goes beyond 30 days.[1] *It is obvious that the longer the cycle the longer is the initial safe period.*

Thus, when the shortest cycle reaches 30 days, the initial period is one of (30 − 19), i.e. 11 days.

One should not, however, abuse this privilege. In fact, in the case of long cycles, as can be judged by the rise in temperature which is always late, ovulation usually occurs late,[2] and this is why the initial period is more important.

It is not, however, impossible, as one may suppose, that this habitual delay in ovulation should diminish sooner or later if the mechanism which promotes the maturation of the ovum resumes its normal function. Ovulation will then draw nearer to the beginning of the cycle, and the initial period as previously determined is no longer safe, especially in its last days.

In order, therefore, to avoid risk, the extra days provided by long cycles should be used with caution. One could be satisfied with the period of 11 days, corresponding to a cycle of 30 days, even if the shortest cycle previously observed has lasted longer than 30 days.

Irregular Cycle.—Even in the case of an irregular cycle, that is to say one whose length varies appreciably from one time to another, it is possible to make use of the temperature curve; the advantage of which lies precisely in such a situation.

---

[1] It is usually said of such a cycle that it is "retarded"; in the sense that the menses appear each time at a date more or less later than the preceding month.

[2] In fact, as the luteal phase cannot last longer than 16 days, a cycle can only be prolonged at the expense of the follicular phase, which implies a delay in ovulation.

The irregularity of a cycle is generally due to the fact that ovulation takes place at a variable date. But the temperature curve follows these variations step by step, and affords automatic protection, if intercourse takes place only after the thermal rise.

It therefore suffices to keep to the general rule: after making use of the period at the beginning of the cycle (calculated according to the shortest cycle), one waits for the thermal rise. *The only difference is that the length of the waiting period may vary from one cycle to another.* But obviously, *one must know how to wait*, and to continue to abstain so long as one has not observed the appearance of the thermal plateau, even if it is late in appearing.

Generally speaking, the irregular cycles are those in which ovulation is always late but with a more or less marked delay at each cycle, as can be seen by the thermal rise which is found to occur more or less later at each time. It follows that the menses themselves are more or less delayed.

Each time that this delay is sufficiently marked, the problem of pregnancy may arise, and women who are afflicted with this type of cycle pass anxious days, which sends them off periodically in a hurry to their doctor, and does not conduce to harmonious relations at home.

Such cases reflect the triumph of the temperature curve, which substitutes for this anxiety a feeling of security, and a knowledge of oneself, resulting in a marital life freed from obsessions. Whatever the delay, there will be no need to fuss if the temperature has not yet shifted, or if it has been noticed that, the rise having been late, the crucial interval of 16 days has not yet elapsed (see p. 40). It will even be possible to foretell the date of onset of menstruation, which will be 10 to 12 days after the beginning of the thermal plateau. Apart from the practical value of knowing beforehand the time of onset of the menses, the accuracy with which it is possible to deduce this, when it would seem hardly possible to do any such thing, will not fail to increase one's confidence in the scientific value of the method.

Much more rarely, *it may happen that ovulation occurs in a completely anarchic manner*, sometimes delayed, which results in a long cycle, sometimes in advance, which results in a short, even a very short, cycle, if ovulation happens prematurely before the 10th day of the cycle, as is occasionally observed at the premenopausal period of life.

In these cases, because of short cycles, the initial period may be reduced, or even abolished if the cycles are very short.

But in all cases the thermal curve makes it possible to safeguard the post-ovulation safe period, to which it may be necessary to restrict intercourse.

Finally, the irregularity of a cycle may be due to the fact that it does not include ovulation: we have seen that in the absence of the element of regulation provided by the corpus luteum, the cycle may show any length (see p. 33). Its duration may therefore vary each time and the anovular cycle then manifests itself as an irregular one.

Anovular Cycle.—The anovular cycle poses a special problem from the point of view of periodic abstention.

It will be recalled that in this type of cycle the temperature remains always at the same level. Therefore, after having made use of the initial safe period, it will not be seen to rise. In conformity with the principles of this method, *intercourse must not be resumed*.

Only at the end of the cycle will it be evident that there has been no rise in temperature; that therefore *it was* a question of an anovular cycle. One will, therefore, have refrained for nothing, since in the absence of ovulation there was no possibility of fertilization in this cycle. But this restraint is necessary, because so long as the temperature has not risen one cannot tell whether ovulation will not occur in the days following.

Naturally, this standpoint will only be justified if cycles which still include ovulation are alternating with those which are anovular, as may happen especially at the pre-menopausal period.

When all cycles are anovular the problem does not arise, since women who show this type of cycle are sterile, and indeed often consult their doctors about remedying this state of affairs. Besides, continued anovular cycles often end up in complete cessation of menstruation.

THE CYCLO-THERMIC CHART

WE have seen that it is necessary to use a special chart or graph, and the following model is proposed (Fig. 17).[1]

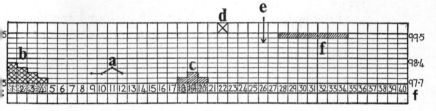

FIG. 17: *Cyclo-thermic chart*

The numbers at the bottom of the chart indicate *the days of the cycle*; the first day, at the extreme left, corresponding to the date of onset of menstruation.

Below this number will be found an empty square which is to be used for the *corresponding day of the month*.

When the next menses start, the chart is changed: thus there is a direct picture of the cycle, the length of which is indicated by the number at the extreme right of the chart which has just been finished.

The temperature is marked on the horizontal line by a dot, corresponding with the figure observed, to be placed in the middle of the vertical column corresponding to the date on which it has been taken (Fig. 17a) (and not at the intersection of the horizontal and vertical lines, or one would not know which day it refers to).

[1] See p. 75 for two cyclo-thermic charts ready for use.

F   67

This chart also makes it possible to note all information which may be useful for the medical study of the cycle.

To indicate *menstruation*, the square for each day on which it has occurred should be filled in with red pencil, and, above this square, as many little squares as will indicate that bleeding has been abundant (Fig. 17b). The same should be done of any *abnormal bleeding* (Fig. 17c).

At the upper part of the chart will be found another row of empty squares. Here one should put in whatever *symptoms* have been noticed, such as congestion of the breasts, pain, etc., and these can be shown by some conventional sign such as a cross (Fig. 17d).

One should also mark with a vertical arrow the column corresponding to those dates on which analyses, examinations, injections, etc., have been carried out (Fig. 17e).

If any medicine is taken over several days, this can be indicated if necessary by shading, as in Fig. 17f.

Thus every symptom, examination, investigation, treatment or incident occurring during the cycle can be noted down on the cyclo-thermic chart at its own date and situated in relation to the thermal curve at that moment.

In this way the doctor will have all possible information before him which, added to a clinical examination, will enable him to establish the diagnosis, formulate the treatment, and check its results.

We should add that, thanks to the thermal chart, *this medical supervision can even be carried out at a distance, by correspondence.*

It often happens that the information gained by repeated clinical examinations as to the condition of the ovaries or the womb does not vary from one time to another. What does change, however, is the menses, cycle, temperature, symptoms felt by the patient; all of which are items of information which it is possible to note accurately on the chart. Following a preliminary clinical examination, therefore, it is possible to follow by means of the chart sent by post the changes in the cycle, the temperature curve, etc., following some prescribed treatment, and thus modify instructions as required.

The opportunity thus afforded to a doctor to follow his patients at a distance, particularly useful in case of absence, is one of the most practical applications of the thermal curve.

CONCLUSION

WITH these last instructions we reach the end of our enterprise, which was to give to every woman the means of knowing and controlling her sexual life.

Casting a backward glance we feel tempted to derive some legitimate satisfaction from it : the world of womanhood, hitherto so mysterious, begins to clear. The menstrual cycle is no longer subject to an obscure mechanism which had to be endured without understanding. We are now able to follow and to explain the variations which seemed to be ordered by pure chance; equally we can follow and recognize ovulation, the presence of the corpus luteum, and the onset of a fresh pregnancy.

To penetrate the secret life of woman, jealously guarded by taboos and interdicts, we have only needed to be able to interpret a simple and banal sign : the temperature !

One might well be surprised that the importance and significance of this sign should have remained unsuspected for so long; that it is only in the last few years that its importance has been realized.

The explanation of this is to be found in the nature of medical science itself. Medicine, a science of correlations, begins the moment when two signs which have been observed with the required exactness can then be related one to another. For example, the observation that a patient has fever or has a yellow complexion does not constitute an advance unless one can relate these observations to another facet of the illness, if one does not know what underlies this fever, this jaundice. Put in another way, it means that there is no medical science unless one can parallel on the one hand the clinical signs observed at the bedside with, on the other, the internal changes in the organs. Another example would be the knowledge that we now have as to the well-recognized "murmur" or sound manifested by a cardiac or pulmonary lesion. When the physician hears such a sound by auscultation, he can deduce the nature of the lesion. This is what, in medical terms, constitutes a *diagnosis*.

This correlation between clinical signs and ana-tomical changes which has issued in the art of medical diagnosis marks a stage in medical evolution which can be termed "anatomo-clinical". It is this method, ren-dered illustrious by the great clinicians of the nine-teenth century, which has laid down the bases of modern medicine, and made possible the great advances which we are now witnessing in all its branches.

In our day this method is still the necessary founda-tion of medical science, but the subsequent progress in techniques of investigation have perfected and refined it, by making it possible to perceive the anatomical lesions themselves. Thus, by means of radiology it is possible to "see" a pulmonary lesion, to confront this knowledge with the signs found on auscultation, and thus verify the diagnostic value of these signs. More-over, thanks to these new techniques, it is possible to discover a lesion at an early stage, before the appearance of external signs which reveal its presence. Thus one can discover by radiological investigation the presence of lesions which are as yet "dumb" from the clinical angle.

It must be realized, however, that the presence of an anatomical lesion implies that the illness is already in an advanced state. Often enough, in fact, an organic lesion is but the end result of a functional disorder. The tendency in modern medicine is to try and discover disturbances of function before they lead to an organic lesion. Correlations now have to be sought, not merely between clinical signs and anatomical lesions, but between these signs and disorders of function which it is now possible to discern and to explain by means of various techniques: physical, chemical, or biological, which are every day more numerous and refined.

Knowledge about the temperature curve in woman first went through the clinical stage, thus following the general line of medical evolution. It had been noted that the temperature rose during the premenstrual period, but in the absence of methods of control, and in the absence of sufficient knowledge about ovarian functions, it was not possible to understand the significance of this sign.[1]

Matters remained at this stage until a new technique made it possible to remove fragments of the uterine mucous membrane and to recognize, microscopically, certain cellular changes brought about by the hormones of the corpus luteum. Thanks to this technique, which is linked with the name of Moricard, the French gynaecologist Raoul Palmer was able to demonstrate some twenty years ago that the premenstrual rise in temperature was associated with the impregnation of the uterine mucosa by the hormones of the corpus luteum and, consequently, that this rise in temperature witnessed the activity of the corpus luteum. So, by this

---

[1] This premenstrual fever was considered to be a sign of latent tuberculosis. But in 1929 the French obstetrician Fruhinsholz of Nancy, describing the raised temperature in the beginning of pregnancy, associated this with premenstrual rise, and, with admirable prescience, formulated the hypothesis that in both cases it was a sign of activity in the corpus luteum.

observation, Palmer laid down in the course of a few years the bases of our knowledge as to the medical usage of the temperature curve; which can truly be said to constitute one of our basic concepts of gynaecology.

A last stage was reached within the past few years with the invention, notably by Marrian and others in England, Venning and Brown in the United States, Max Jayle in France, of chemical techniques which made it possible to gain a direct measurement of the hormones of the corpus luteum, or of its decomposition products in the urine. There was now a direct and indisputable index of the activity of the corpus luteum, thanks to which it was now possible to control the reliability of the information given by the temperature curve. This study confirmed the previous conclusions by making them more precise, and it can now be affirmed that the thermal curve is a very faithful reflection of the activities of the corpus luteum.[1]

But there is more to it: by making it possible to study separately the different hormonal activities of the corpus luteum and measuring them, these methods help in the total understanding of ovarian function. They also make it possible to detect ovarian disorders at a very early stage indeed—while these are still reversible by appropriate treatment—and even before any clinical manifestation, as we have seen to be the case in the preventive supervision of pregnancy from the endocrine angle.

Let us add that, as they complete the information derived from the temperature curve, these techniques also furnish a means of establishing the limits of the thermal method: one should not expect from it more information than it can give, which is to register the presence of the corpus luteum and to indicate the duration of its functional activity.

[1] See Appendix, p. 78.

This brief incursion into the philosophy of medicine has shown us that the temperature curve, far from being an empirical method or a mere practical formula, is a part of the evolution of medical science, and that it rests on scientific findings which are among the most firmly established in the experimental field.

Except for those who remain invincibly ignorant, it would appear that these are sufficient arguments to persuade all those gifted with reason not to deprive themselves of the material and moral advantages to be gained by the use of the temperature curve.

Use this page for your first two months' charts.

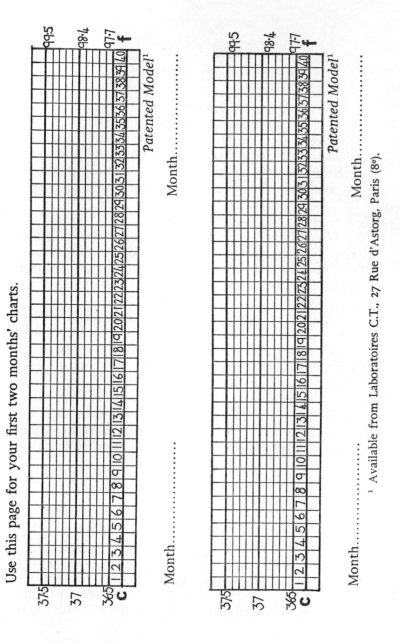

Month........

Month........

Patented Model[1]

Month........

Month........

Patented Model[1]

[1] Available from Laboratoires C.T., 27 Rue d'Astorg, Paris (8e).

APPENDIX

We wish to add here some extra instructions, chiefly meant for medical readers, who might be called upon to give advice on the subject of temperatures. We shall do so in the form of the three following notes: one relating to a special use of the temperature, the others to some objections on principle which demand a reply.

Note 1

The thermal curve, which has helped us up to now only to determine the post-ovulation safe period, *can also be used with advantage instead of the Ogino-Knaus calculation in order to determine the first or initial safe period.*

Though the thermal curve cannot indicate in advance what *will be* the date of ovulation during the current cycle, it can tell us what *was* the actual date on which ovulation occurred in past cycles. By examining all the curves during the year which has gone by, one can determine *the date of the earliest ovulation* hitherto observed. It will then be sufficient to subtract from this date the two days during which the sperm can survive and one extra day "for protection" in order to obtain the initial period which can be made use of.

Example: If the study of previous curves shows that the earliest ovulation took place on the 12th day of the cycle, the 11th and 10th days must be excluded, and also the 9th, giving an initial period of 8 days.

The initial period calculated in this way is usually more favourable than that by the Ogino-Knaus method. The latter, which is based on the shortest cycle observed hitherto, only takes count of the total length of the cycle and necessarily ignores the mechanism which may shorten it.[1] This is a blind calculation and may have the effect of diminishing or even suppressing the initial sterile period in a case where this need not be necessary.

Given a cycle of 28 days which is accidentally shortened to 23 days, the Ogino-Knaus calculation would indicate that the initial period should be reduced to (23 − 19), i.e. 4 days. Let us now suppose that the thermal curve has shown that in fact this 23-day cycle corresponds to an ovulation on the 12th day, followed by a corpus luteum of 11 days. Thanks to the thermal curve one can now use an initial period corresponding to an ovulation on the 12th day; that is to say, 8 days, as we have seen, instead of only 4.

This use of the temperature curve is of particular interest to those who are afflicted by a short cycle, where the security afforded by the Ogino-Knaus calculation is too dearly obtained by an excessive reduction in the length of the initial safe period.

All the same, it is important to stress that *the use of the thermal curve in this way implies complete ability to recognize ovulation on this curve*, whereas we have seen that this is in no way necessary with the habitual use of the curve, where it is sufficient to recognize that the temperature has been stabilized at the higher level.

Now, to recognize ovulation on the curve requires considerable familiarity with thermal charts. It is in fact a medical diagnosis. For this reason we think that *this special use of the thermal curve should be reserved for doctors.*[2]

[1] Which may be due to advanced ovulation, but also to a shortened duration of the corpus luteum, or indeed to an association of the two factors.

[2] All the more because the thermal curve does not always enable one to recognize the exact day of ovulation; the precise diagnosis of which demands the use of more elaborate methods such as vaginal smears, hormone analysis, etc.

Note 2

We wish now to reply to certain objections on matters of principle which are often raised, according to which the phenomena of life are too varied, too rich, to be encompassed in their totality; that exceptions are always possible, which may upset any method.

Thus, while recognizing the validity of the thermal curve as a test of luteal activity, one might tend to accord it only a statistical significance, pointing out that it may prove false in a not inconsiderable number of cases. In fact, as pointed out by certain authors[1] and as confirmed by modern methods of hormonal investigation, it may happen that the temperature does not rise in spite of the presence of a corpus luteum, the activity of which is shown by the normality of hormone elimination.

These cases, which are exceedingly rare, are to be explained by an absence of sensitivity on the part of the thermo-regulating centres to the hormone of the corpus luteum. But even though one cannot deny the existence of such cases, though it is important to note their extreme rarity, it must be emphasized that they in no way threaten the use of the method of the safe period, since this implies abstention so long as the temperature remains low.

On the other hand one can rest assured that *there is no thermal plateau without a corpus luteum.* Hence, and for the reasons already given, which prevent the onset of a second ovulation, *one can be absolutely certain* that intercourse at the time of the thermal plateau cannot be followed by pregnancy.[2]

[1] Siegler (S. L.) and Siegler (A. M.), *Evaluation of the Basal Body Temperature, Fertility and Sterility,* 1951, 2, 287.

[2] The possibility of a second ovulation has been discussed, though it is very questionable. What may possibly happen is that after an abortive ovulation, not followed by a corpus luteum, a second ovulation may occur, this one actually fol-

To sum up, despite the possibility of a dissociation such as we have indicated above, we can agree with Netter who states: "In general the thermal curve, so far as the recognition of the presence or absence of the corpus luteum is concerned, has great value, and a degree of accuracy greater than the vast majority of biological tests."[1]

Note 3

Inspired by this same notion, that the richness and complexity of life will render calculation vain and negate all previsions, some people would deny that there is any security about the first sterile period because, theoretically, an ovulation may occur which is sooner than the earliest one observed previously.

Such an attitude springs from a narrow and mistaken attitude towards science. Carried to the extreme, it would lead to a negation of all biological science and, therefore, of the whole medical art itself. To reason in this way is to import into the sciences of life concepts which are only valid in the so-called "exact" sciences; an attitude which is even less justifiable now that we have reached a stage when in Physics itself the convictions of yesterday are changed into truths in which the calculus of probability and the laws for great numbers take first place.

[1] Netter (A.) and others, "Fonction lutéale et courbe ménothermique" in *Colloques sur la Fonction lutéale*, Masson éd., Paris, 1953, Vol. I, p. 315.

---

lowed by a normally active corpus luteum. But the first ovulation, not being followed by a corpus luteum, does not evoke a thermal plateau, which appears only after the secondary ovulation. This occurrence, therefore, does not at all impair the method. Besides, these facts are so exceptional, if they exist at all, that they do not deserve to be taken into account in practice.

Can one say, however, that this objection has no foundation? Certainly not. But if we must recognize its validity we must also be prepared to measure its limits and take into account its relative nature.

The biologists, relying on a great number of observations, are at one in affirming that premature ovulations starting before the 10th day of the cycle are quite exceptional, that, moreover, these produce ova which are insufficiently mature, so that their chances of fertilization are practically nil. Still, a strictly reasoned argument might insist that the possibility of fertilization is theoretically possible.

Contrary to some opinions, the contradiction between these two propositions is not so extreme as would appear. In practice, in the case of a woman whose genital function is normal, the chances that ovulation might extend beyond the limits set by the calculation, and would result in pregnancy, are very faint, and it would be unjustifiable to deprive oneself of the initial safe period, having regard to the minimal risk. The same does not apply, however, where the cycle is very irregular, or in a pre-menopausal state; in such a case the risk of premature ovulation must not be neglected and a prudent attitude would be justified (see p. 65).

Conclusion: The fact that the safe period at the beginning of the cycle cannot, *in theory*, be considered *perfectly safe*, does not imply that, *in practice*, it has no security at all: "absence of complete security" is not the same as "complete absence of security".

There is indeed a *hierarchy in security*, which is all the greater as the initial period is more strictly calculated; this security becoming absolute when intercourse is limited to the phase of post-ovulation, this being always possible with the thermal curve, in any circumstance.

Thanks to the understanding of the mechanism of the

cycle furnished by the thermal curve, we are now in a position to appreciate the risk to be taken in any particular case according to the initial period which it is decided to make use of. It follows that a subtle use of this initial period will be possible, and it is for each to decide, according to one's instinct, personality and feeling at the moment, the degree of risk which one is prepared to run.[1]

[1] For those who would feel paralysed by having to make too great a decision, let us recall the fact that the method of calculating the initial period offers a very wide margin of safety indeed.